A S...

Homeopathic Philosophy

R. Gibson Miller
M.D.

REVISED AND ENLARGED

by

James Tyler Kent
M.D.

B. Jain Publishers (P) Ltd.

An ISO 9001 : 2000 Certified Company
USA – Europe – India

A Synopsis

of

HOMEOPATHIC PHILOSOPHY

Revised Edition: 2007

Published by Kuldeep Jain for

B. Jain Publishers (P) Ltd.

An ISO 9001 : 2000 Certified Company
1921, Street No. 10, Chuna Mandi, Paharganj
New Delhi 110 055 (INDIA)
Ph. 91-11-2358 0800, 2358 3100, 2358 1300, 2358 1100
Fax: 91-11-2358 0471
E-mail: bjain@vsnl.com
Website: www.bjainbooks.com

Printed in India by :
Akash Press, New Delhi-110020.

BOOK CODE / ISBN: 978-81-319-0174-8

Introduction

Feeling the necessity of having in a concise
and accessible form the various sub-laws and
rules of homeopathy, I prepared for my own
use the following arrangement of them.
Dr. Kent very kindly revised the
manuscript and made a number
of valuable additions, and also
suggested that it might be of
service to others if
published.

R. Gibson Miller

CONTENTS

CLASSIFICATION OF DISEASES

All non-surgical diseases belong to one of the following classes: (a) Acute; (b) Chronic; (c) Those due to the use of drugs, living under unhealthy conditions, etc.

Acute Diseases

1. Acute diseases are self-limited, and provided no treatment is pursued, they end in resolution or death.

   This being so an acute disease can have no sequelae, the so called sequelae being manifestations of one of the chronic miasms roused into activity by the acute disease.

2. Acute diseases may be stopped at any stage by the similar remedy.

3. In acute infectious diseases all infection ceases as soon as the simillimum is given.

4. The best prophylactic in acute disease is the epidemic remedy.

5. When a trivial acute disease supervenes during the treatment of a chronic one, it is advisable to use the indicated remedy in a low potency; for, if this is done, it will often be found after the acute disease has been cured, that the deep-acting remedy has not been interfered with by the short acting one, and that it still continues to act.

   (This is unlikely if the acute disease is severe. If it is severe acute disease, don't expect this, and give the remedy in potency. — J.T. Kent)

6. After the cure of the *acute supervening* disease it is advisable, before repeating the remedy for the chronic disease, to make sure that the chronic disease has not been modified by the treatment of the acute one, or by the acute disease itself, and not to call for a different remedy from that formerly needed.

7. When the acute disease has been modified by allopathic or inappropriate homeopathic

remedies, it is usually advisable to prescribe for the case as it now stands, rather than according to the original symptoms.

8. *Acute* exacerbations of *active chronic* disease must be treated in a different way from that of an acute supervening disease, provided any remedy is required at all. Frequently the acute complement of the deep-acting remedy, required by the chronic disease is the suitable one, but if only an antipsoric is called for it is better not to give any medicine.

9. Commonly, when the chronic disease is only partially active, as shown by the patient being apparently in good health except that slight causes give rise to frequent acute attacks of illness, the knowledge of the remedy for these acute manifestations will enable us to select its complementary deep-acting remedy, and so permit the cure of the chronic underlying disease.

Chronic Diseases

1. Chronic diseases are characterized by their progressing from without inwards and from below upwards, and, that while the symptoms may vary, they never disappear in the reverse order to that in which they came.

2. So far as it at present known there are only three chronic diseases, viz., psora, syphilis and sycosis.

   These diseases may be active or latent.

   They may be present in three ways, viz. :

   (a) A single miasm.

   (b) Two or three miasms co-existing, but separate and only one active at a time.

   (c) Two or three of the miasms may form a complex and this may be further complicated by a drug disease.

   If two or more miasms from a complex, the proper remedy will dissociate them, and then the most active must be attacked; but the greatest caution is needed, as a mistake may cause them again to combine, and they will never again separate.

3. These chronic diseases often remain latent for long periods, but are apt to be roused into activity by acute diseases, unhealthy surroundings, grief, etc.

   While latent their symptoms are very similar, and the patient may only feel ill in an indefinite way.

   The nosodes of these diseases are frequently of great service in rationalizing the symptoms of such cases, and thus enabling the appropriate remedy to be found.

4. These diseases are always taken at the stage in which they exist in the already infected person. For example, the wife of a man with secondary syphilis will take the disease at that stage and not in the primary or chancre stage.-[Kent in *Journal of homeopathics*, March, 1899.]

5. A man with syphilis or sycosis may fail to infect his wife if she is suffering from some other but dissimilar, protecting, chronic diseases such as

phthisis, for dissimilar diseases repel one another.

THE TOTALITY OF THE SYMPTOMS

As our sole guide in the choice of the curative remedy is the totality of the symptoms, it is necessary to enquire what is meant by the totality.

In acute disease every symptom experienced by the patient or observable by others is to be included in the totality; also any cause, such as wetting, fright, etc., and circumstances aggravating and ameliorating.

As an acute disease never forms a *complex* with a chronic one, the latter being suppressed until the former one has run its course, care must be taken when ascertaining the symptoms of the acute disease not to take into account old symptoms which belong to the chronic disease. But in some cases of acute disease, SYMPTOMS of the chronic disease remain, and are active during the acute disease; such chronic *symptoms* are peculiar because they have not disappeared, and very often are guiding to the cure of the acute disease; while the remedy will have no relation to the chronic disease, yet that peculiar symptom will stand out and guide you to the remedy that will cure the acute disease, such symptoms are peculiar to the patient [Kent, *Medical Advance*, January 1890.]

In chronic disease the toatality includes all symptoms experienced by the patient since birth, excluding those arising during acute disease. While theoretically it is proper to include all such symptoms yet great caution must be used. (1) some other chronic miasm may have been acquired during life, or (2) the symptoms may have been so perverted by inappropriate treatment that they do not truly represent the disease- (Kent, *Journal of Homeopathics* July 1899.) When the symptoms have been much perverted by inappropriate treatment we can sometime get a sure foundation on which to base a prescription by taking the symptoms as experienced by the patient before this inappropriate treatment was commenced.

This investigation into the former symptoms of the patient is frequently of great service when the presently existing symptoms do not point clearly to any remedy. For example, in an adult with neuralgia of the limbs, where present symptoms are not guiding, if we find that in infancy he had scaldhead like that of *Mez.*, and we now examine the neuralgias produced by that remedy, it will often be found that they bear a close resemblance to that of the patient, and it will probably prove curative and reproduce the original eruption.

It frequently happens that, when we search for the totality of the symptoms, we find they have been so perverted or suppressed by inappropriate treatment that those now present do not present a true picture of the internal disease. For example, take a case of gonorrhea suppressed by *Arg- n.*, and on examination there will be found a pretty full picture of *Med.* and a partial one of *Arg- n.* and probably *Nat- m.*

[In all such cases we must prescribe upon the symptoms if possible, but if the case dose not respond and the suppressing drug is known, it is sometimes advisable to select a remedy competing which has an antidotal relationship.-Kent]

In determining the totality, especially with regard to former symptoms in chronic disease, it is also necessary to ascertain whether *one or more miasms* are present, as it is useless to attempt to find a remedy for all the symptoms when there is more than one. In such cases, as a *rule*, only one miasm is active at a time, and the treatment must be directed against that one. When two or more miasms form a complex we must endeavour to separate them.

[The symptoms are the only guide to the separating of the miasms. The road to death is by more complexity and any remedy that improves the patient will cause a simplification or separation of the miasms. -Kent.]

THE SELECTION OF THE REMEDY

Having, then, determined the totality of the symptoms, we must now search for the remedy that has produced symptoms most similar to those observed in the patient. Theoretically we endeavour to discover a remedy whose symptoms exactly correspond in character and grade to those of the patient; but this can rarely if ever be done, and accordingly Hahnemann directs that in searching for the homeopathic specific remedy we ought to be particularly and almost exclusively attentive to the symptoms that are *striking*, *singular, extraordinary* and *peculiar (characteristic)*.

It is especially those symptoms that are *peculiar to the patient* and not to the disease, that are to be our guides. For example, the characteristics of dysentery are bloody discharges, pain and tenesmus; but if fainting accompanied every stool, that would be peculiar to the patient, not to the disease, and hence guiding.

In determining what are characteristic symptoms of the case the following rules and cautions are of importance, viz. :

1. The characteristic symptoms must be equally well marked, both in the patient and in the remedy. In other words, no matter how peculiar a symptom may be, either in the patient or in the remedy, unless it is distinctive and outstanding we must pay little heed to it.

2. No one symptom, however, peculiar it may be, can be our true guide, for, unless there is a general correspondence between the symptoms of the patient and the remedy, failure will result. Those single peculiar symptoms are however, invaluable in suggesting special remedies as

being worthy of examination.

3. General symptoms, or those that effect the whole body, are of very much higher rank than particulars which only relate to special organs; so much so that any number of particular symptoms can be overruled by one strong general.

What the patient predicates of himself is usually general, as when he says, "I am thirsty", meaning that his whole body is so and not any one special organ.

General symptoms, however, are of different grades of value. In the highest rank must be placed all mental symptoms, if at all well marked, and of these all symptoms of the will and affections, including desires and aversions, also irritability and sadness, are the most important. Of less importance are disorders of the intelligence, while those of memory rank lowest of the mental symptoms.

Amongst general symptoms are to be included those in connection with sleep, dreams, the menstrual state, also, the effects of the whether and sensitiveness of the patient to heat and cold.

The special senses are so closely related to the whole man that their symptoms are often general. For example, when a patient says the smell of food sickens him it is a general symptom, whereas an imaginary bad smell in the nose should be particular.

We frequently find on examining the particular organs that some symptom or modality runs strongly through them all, and may be predicated of person himself, so that here we have a general made up of a series of particulars.

4. Care must be taken not to mistake a modality for a symptom, yet circumstances affecting many symptoms become leading characteristics of the patient and hence are important.

5. The skin being the outermost part will yield the least important symptoms.

6. In organic diseases and in many affections of the female genitals we can place little reliance on the local symptoms.

7. A tumor or other pathological condition is no guide to the curative remedy; for in the first place it is not the disease itself, but its result,

and in the second place proving have been pushed far enough to produce similar conditions.

PATHOLOGY

While we must ignore pathological changes when choosing the remedy, yet a knowledge of true pathology is absolutely necessary.

1. We can only thereby understand the course and progress of the case.

2. We can thereby know the symptoms that are common to that special state, and hence those that are peculiar to the patient.

3. We also thereby know in certain diseases, or at certain stages of diseases, that no matter how similar the symptoms produced by some remedies may appear to those of the patient, yet, owing to the superficial character of their action, they cannot prove curative. For example, in pneumonia, in the stage of exudation, while the symptoms may apparently call for *Acon.*, we know that remedy cannot

produce such a condition, and closer examination will reveal that some deeper-acting remedy, such as *Sulph.* or *Lyc.*, is needed.

4. Pathology enables us to decide, when new symptoms arise, whether they are due to the natural progress of the disease or to the action of the remedy.

5. We must clearly understand that it is the patient that is curable and not the disease, and without a proper understanding of pathology we are liable to err. Suppose a case of inflammation of a joint that has led to ankylosis. The suitable remedy will cure the inflammation, but will be powerless to break down the adhesions and surgical aid must be sought. The same holds good with regard to tumors, for when the patient is cured the tumor will ceases to grow; and perhaps it may be absorbed, but very often it persists and must be removed by the knife.

6. Pathology also warns us that it is dangerous to attempt to cure certain conditions of disease,

such as advanced tubercular phthisis, or where foreign bodies are encysted near vital organs. In such cases nature can only cure by suppurating out such foreign substances, and the exhaustion entailed by such an operation is often fatal.

CONCOMITANT SYMPTOMS

It is mistake to suppose that a remedy can cure groups of symptoms only in the order in which they appear in the proving. Often a remedy cures a group whose component parts were observed in different provers and often in quite a different order.

While this is so, experience teaches that certain groups of symptoms are apt to appear together, and when this is so they are more characteristic of the remedy.

Hering says that comparative value of concomitants may be determined thus. If they are essentially concomitant, one being really the cause of the other (*e.g.*, lachrymation due to a general catarrhal condition), then this feature of the case must be considered, but if no such relation of cause and effect is observed it may be ignored.

EFFECTS PRODUCED BY THE REMEDY

The remedy having been given it will affect the case in one of the following ways :

1. The remedy causes no change-either the remedy or the potency in incorrect.

2. Steady rapid improvement takes place without any aggravation.

   (a) In such rapid cases the remedy and potency have been exactly similar to the disease force.

   (b) It may also mean that the disease has not been deeply rooted.

N.B. : There may be an almost complete removal of the symptoms, yet if the patient is not conscious of the elasticity of returning health it has been no cure, but only palliation.

3. A sharp short aggravation followed by quick improvement and in this case the improvement is usually long lasting.

4. A long aggravation and final slow improvement.

   This occurs chiefly in weakly patients, and there is great danger in repeating the remedy too soon.

5. A long aggravation, followed by slow decline of the patient.

   These cases are incurable and only short-acting remedies should be used.

6. A sharp aggravation, but the improvement that follows is very lasting, especially when a deep-acting remedy has been given.
   These cases are usually incurable.

7. Rapid improvement but soon followed by an aggravation.

   If the remedy was the *simillimum* the case is incurable, but if the remedy only corresponded superficially it may have acted palliatively.

8. The amelioration lasts a normal time, but a new group of symptoms appear and under another suitable remedy they disappear for the normal time and another new group of symptoms appear, yet, in spite of the removal of group

after group, the patient steadily declines. This is especially observed in the old and feeble and such cases are incurable.

9. New symptoms appear (not the return of old ones which have been experienced long before the remedy was given).

   (*a*) If the new symptoms belong to the pathogenesis of the remedy the remedy is the correct one, and must be allowed to act. If the new symptoms are not known to belong to the pathogenesis of the remedy and yet the case rapidly improves, it is probable that further provings will show that they really do belong to it.

   (*b*) If the new symptoms are due to the natural development of the disease, then probably the remedy has been wrong and has produced no effect.

   These new symptoms may be due, however, to a natural crisis of the disease, such as epistaxis in typhus, and must not be interfered with.

(*c*) If the new symptoms, though numerous and violent, do not belong to the natural development of the disease (and the patient does not improve), then the remedy is the wrong one.

10. An aggravation followed by the return of old symptoms. This is a very favourable state of affairs, and must not be interfered with, for no remedy is homeopathic to reaction. When the symptoms finally settle, if these old symptoms still persist, they must then be prescribed for, and are of the highest grade in the choice of next remedy.

11. There is improvement, but it takes the wrong direction. For example, an ulcer of the leg heals up under the action of the remedy, but hemorrhage from the lungs comes on. This shows that the remedy only corresponded to part of the case, viz., the ulcer, and has really done harm.

12. In some patient we get a proving of every remedy given. They are oversensitive and very difficult to cure.

THE HOMEOPATHIC AGGRAVATION

In acute diseases the homeopathic aggravation is not, as a rule, marked unless the disease has been severe and dangerous.

In chronic cases *without* tissue changes the aggravation is usually not severe, but when there are tissue changes there is almost invariably a marked aggravation usually with elimination through some of the natural orifices of the body.

In the former the aggravation is due to the medicinal disease, where as in the latter it is due to an effort on nature's part to put matters right-a sort of house cleaning.

When the remedy does not correspond exactly to the disease symptoms we are not likely to have an aggravation (except in over-sensitives, where it is medicinal and not curative).

This is especially observable in feeble patients who, owing to their deficient vitality, are not able to produce any guiding symptoms. [Kent, *Journal of Homeopathics*, May 1900.]

THE REPETITION OF THE REMEDY

The medicine must not be repeated until the action of the last dose is fully exhausted. In other words, there can be no fixed time as to when to repeat, each case must be judged on its own merits.

In acute cases it is comparatively easy to determine when the last does has exhausted its action by means of the general appearance and mental state of the patient, and also to a less degree by the pulse and temperature.

In typhoid fever in vigorous patients Kent usually gives the remedy in water every few hours for several days, because it is a continued fever, but on the slightest sign of reaction stops the remedy.

On the other hand, he does *not* repeat the remedy in continued fever in a feeble patient.

In remittent fever reaction will appear in a few hours, and one does is sufficient.

But in chronic cases it is not so easy, *for it is the rule and not the exception to have sharp, short exacerbations interrupting* the improvement, and we must be sure that the exacerbation is a permanent and not a mere passing one.

In chronic cases we know that the dose is still acting as long as old symptoms return, or, if the symptoms continue to disappear in the reverse order to that in which they originally appeared, or if they pass from internal organs to more superficial parts, or if they go from above down.

More cases are spoiled by too frequent repetition then from any other cause, and it must be remembered that an acute case may show no improvement for *three days* and some chronic ones for *sixty*.

When vitality is very low, as in collapse, it is dangerous to repeat the dose. But when there is a lack of response to the remedy after allopathic drugging, which is really due to a sluggishness and not to a want of vitality, it is necessary to repeat often. -[Kent]

Incurable disease requires more frequent repetition of the short acting remedies for palliation and it is advisable to use a higher potency than the 200th. [Kent *Journal of Homeopathics* Nov. 1897.]

Some antipsorics have also an acute action, and when indicated in acute disease behave exactly like the short-acting remedies.

When the remedy corresponds very closely to the disease the symptoms, after a reasonable time, will come back exactly the same or perhaps with the omission of one or two. In such cases all we have to do is repeat the same remedy and potency until it fails to act, when another potency must be used. Unfortunately in chronic diseases it is rarely possible to select a remedy that corresponds with perfect accuracy to the disease, and consequently when the symptoms return they are some-what changed; and frequent repetition of the original remedy will confuse the case, for it is possible to suppress symptoms by the too frequent use of even high potencies.

THE SECOND REMEDY

The first remedy having done all that it can, we must proceed to choose the second one. If the symptoms came in the order a, b, c, d and e, and after a dose of an antipsoric remedy we find great improvement for 6 or 8 weeks, with the disappearance of symptoms e, d, c and then a and b again increase and even e returns, but d and c have permanently gone, finally a new symptom f appears so that we now have a, b, c, f, this last appearing symptom, f, is guiding and will appear in the anamnesis as best related to some medicine which has it as a characteristic. Hering says that this new symptom, f, will generally be found amongst the symptoms of the last given remedy, but only of low rank. It is on account of the appearance of this new symptom and the disappearance of d and e that original remedy is now contraindicated.

The second remedy must *bear a complementary relation to the first*, and hence the last remedy, either homeopathic or allopathic, that has acted forms one of the most important guides in the choice of the second remedy.

If a case has been much drugged we are often forced to give *Nux-v.* as an antidote. This giving of *Nux-v.* however, does not confine our choice of the remedy that is to follow to the 8 or 10 remedies which bear a complementary relation to *Nux-v.* for *Nux-v.* has a wide range and after giving it the case will open up and you can give any remedy excepting *Zinc*, which would have to be avoided.

POTENCY

The minimum dose is as essential to homeopathy as the law of similars.

The best results are only obtained when the disease force and the remedial force are on the same plane. This may explain why in some cases a low potency cures after the failure of a high. When a medicine needs repetition it should be given in the same potency as long as it will act.

If the remedy called for during an acute exacerbation is afterwards needed for the chronic condition it must be given in a different potency.

Very high potencies should not be used in incurable cases.

In certain oversensitive very high potencies instead of curing always cause provings, and such people do better with the 200th or 1M. When the patient has been long accustomed to the use of low potencies you do not always get good results from the higher potencies at first. Conversely the frequent proving of high potencies seems to develop a susceptibility and such provers obtain more and finer symptoms than those who have only proved low potencies.

In all periodic diseases, periodic either with regard to pain, convulsions, or discharges, it is not advisable to give the remedy during the exacerbation but immediately after it. [Kent, *Journal of Homeopathics* Sept. 1897.]

DIRECTION OF SYMPTOMS DURING CURE

1. From within out.
2. Usually from above downwards.
3. In the reverse order to that in which they appeared.

This process goes on until the primary manifestations of the disease appear, whether it be the chancer of syphilis, the gonorrhea of sycosis, or the eruption of psora.

The original discharge may not come back at the original place, but *from* some other mucus membrane. It is also to be remembered that the miasms may be taken at any stage, and consequently if a woman takes syphilis from her husband in the sore throat stage we can only bring back the disease to the point and not to the chancre.

INIMICAL REMEDIES

Remedies which are very similar in action either antidote one another or are inimical. *This latter relation only holds good provided the first given remedy has acted and to some extent influenced the case.* When the first remedy has taken possession, he is the proprietor and this relation should be respected. If the first remedy has had no effect its inimical may be given with perfect safety.

Some remedies are inimical to each other in their acute sphere and others only in their chronic. (Kent, *Med. Adv.*, Jan. 9 1895).

MANAGEMENT OF ABNORMAL CRAVINGS

In acute dises it is advisable to yield to the cravings of the patient, but in chronic disease they must *not* be indulged.

It is to be noted that when a patient has by long continued use becomes habituated to drugs, such as morphia, tobacco, etc., the homeopathic remedy *will at times*, act inspite of the continued use of the drug; but, of course, the action is short-lasting and imperfect.

CAUTIONS TO BE OBSERVED IN THE USE OF CREATAIN REMEDIES

Certain remedies, such as *Sulphur, Silicia Phos.* and *Sul- ac.*, owing to their power of expelling foreign bodies are very dangerous in some diseases, as these bodies can only be got rid of by suppuration. In far advanced phthisis with tubercular deposit or where healing of the diseased part with calcareous deposit has taken place, or when foreign bodies, such as bullets, are encysted near vital organs, this danger is a very real one.

There are two classes of symptoms in all advanced tubercular and suppurative lung diseases, viz. the toxemic and constitutional; the chest pains, the hectic fever, the mental symptoms and dreams being toxemic.

If one of this group of remedies, say *Sil.*, only corresponds to the toxemic symptoms and not to the constitutional ones, it will palliate by subduing the toxemic symptoms without doing any damage.

But, if prior to the formation of the tubercle, the patient suffered from weekly headaches coming up the back of the head, offensive foot sweats, sensitiveness to cold, etc., and though these may have all disappeared even before the phthisis came on, the *Sil.* will prove a most dangerous remedy-[Kent, *Journal of Homeopathics*, Nov. 1899.]

At times these remedies for the same reason are apt to cause damage after hemorrhage into the brain or other important organs.

Ferr. and *Acet-ac.* are dangerous in many cases of advanced phthisis, owning to their power of inducing hemorrhage.

Ferr. in old syphilitics is apt to render ulcers phagedenic.

Antipsorics are apt to do harm in active syphilis, i.e., as long as the syphilis is the uppermost miasm. But many antipsorics are also anti-syphilitics, and they are not to be excluded by the rule.

It is dangerous to stop the diarrhea of advanced phthisis even by the indicated remedy.

Kali- c., is a very dangerous remedy in old gouty cases, but *Kali- i.* is often very beneficial,-(Kent).

Ars. is very dangerous remedy in irritable heart, especially if organic, as it is apt to cause parenchymatous nephritis,-(Kent).

Ars. is dangerous remedy in dysentery if not the exact *simillimum,*as it is very apt to spoil the case-(Kent *Med. Adv.*, Nov. 1899).

IDIOSYNCRASY

Every one has some idiosyncrasy or peculiar susceptibility to certain influences. It is for this reason that only a few persons out of the many are affected when exposed to the infinitesimal noxia that cause disease. The sensitiveness of a sick man to the homeopathic *Simillimum* is wonderful, while a remedy that is not homeopathic to this condition may be given in massive doses with little effect. No one can be made sick in a lasting way by drug to which he is not susceptible. This fact may serve to explain how at times a high potency of the same drug with which a person is poisoned proves curative. In other words, in such a case the patient was poisoned because he was already sick or susceptible and needed that remedy, but the drug not being on the same plane as his susceptibility poisoned instead of curing him.

(Kent also suggests that frequent repetitions of a crude drug may bring about susceptibility to it, and that after a time the merest inhalation of it may produce its effects. (*Hom. Phys.*, Sept., 1889.)

PROVINGS

It is advisable when making provings to begin with a single dose, but in the great majority of cases this will cause no effect. If the single dose fails we may try to create a susceptibility by repeating the dose until some effect is produced, but the medicine must be stopped at once on the appearance of symptoms and not repeated until absolutely all symptoms have ceased.

Many provings, especially some of *Thuja.*, are almost valueless owing to this repetition of the drug after symptoms appeared. The finest symptoms, as a rule, are those that develop late, months after the drug has been discontinued. No heed must be paid as to whether the symptoms in a proving are primary or secondary, for as long as the drug can produce them it can cure them. In certain provers what are commonly regarded as secondary symptoms appear as the primary action of the drug.

In a proving, if symptoms appear which have been experienced long before, this re-appearance only proves that in virtue of his own constitution this prover has a special tendency to admit their manifestation.-[*Organon*, par. 138.]

PSORA

In the treatment of chronic non-veneral disease Hahnemann found that the similar remedy was just as efficacious in removing the existing symptoms as it was in acute disease. But he also frequently found that while the patient might remain well for a considerable period, yet without adequate cause the same symptoms returned and where again removed by the remedy, though less perfectly than before. This happened several times, until finally the remedy ceased to benefit.

Being convinced of the universality of the homeopathic law of cure, he concluded that the ostensible disease could not be the whole, but only the active part of some much more extensive disease, or otherwise it would have been permanently cured.

Accordingly he endeavoured by careful examination of the history and progress of a large number of chronic diseases to discover all the ailments and symptoms belonging to this unknown primitive malady. He found that the majority of such patients had the itch or some other cutaneous disease, such as eczema, herpes, tinea, etc., and that the symptoms of the chronic disease only began to manifest themselves after these had disappeared or had been removed by external treatment, and that the disease constantly tended to progress from without inwards from the lesser to the more vitally important organs. Having now, as he believed, discovered the common origin of all the variously named chronic diseases, which he called psora, he chose from amongst the then proven remedies all such as were capable or producing symptoms similar to those of the miasm and advised that they should be employed in its cure.

Hahnemann believed that psora was always the result of direct infection, and probably this was the case originally; but now, according to Kent, all mankind is more or less psoric and the acute manifestation is only the taking on a new load of the disease.

Many have rejected the psora theory, but practical experience teaches us to give by preference these very antipsoric remedies. This preference is not theoretical and is constantly subordinate to the general principles of homeopathy.

Dr. Ruter published what he believed to be the order in which the various organs were affected by psora, when not interfered with, but Kent is unable to confirm this sequence. Kent has observed that many diseases seem to be on the same plane, one member of a family having epilepsy, while others have insanity, cancer, tuberculosis, etc, the various organs being affected according to the circumstances of the patient.

SYPHILIS

The true course of this disease cannot be properly followed from old school writings, as their habitual use of massive doses prevents the disease following its natural course.

The primary manifestation is the chancre, which usually appears fifteen days after exposure. This chancre, under proper homeopathic treatment, tends to enlarge, and the bubo frequently suppurates, whereas, under allopathic treatment, the bubo remains as a hard lump and seldom suppurates. Under homeopathic treatment the bubo disappears if the chancre discharges profusely.

Hahnemann taught that it was possible to prevent the appearance of secondary symptoms, but this is a mistake, for they always sooner or later appear. In Hahnemann's day the distinction between the chancre and chancroid was not properly understood, and doubtless it was this that led him into error. The chancre is followed by the eruptions which likely call for a different remedy. The closer the remedy given for the chancre is to the *simillimum* the less copious will be the eruption.

The eruptions under homeopathic treatment are usually very profuse, but are never pustular. The eruption is followed by ulceration of the throat. The first ulcer to come will be the last to disappear under homeopathic treatment. The next manifestation is the falling out of the hair. [Kent]

The tertiary stage under homeopathic treatment, if it appears at all, is a shadow. [Kent]

The foregoing only holds true when the treatment has been purely homeopathic throughout, but when we are called on to treat a case that has passed down to the tertiary stage under allopathic treatment the procedure is very different.

In such a case under appropriate treatment all the symptoms he has already experienced will return, but in the opposite order to which they originally appeared, viz., the falling out of the hair, then the sore throat eruptions and finally the chancre. Of course, these various stages will call for different remedies according to the symptoms, (Never leave *Merc.* So long as it benefits, Kent)

Syphilis, like sycosis, is always taken at the stage it is in the person from whom it is caught, and consequently when under homeopathic treatment the symptoms begin to come back in the reverse order- they go back to the stage at which the patient took the disease. In old broken down syphilitics without any very guiding symptoms it is advisable to give a few doses of *Syphilinum*, which usually serves to re-establish the vital reaction and bring out the symptoms. After *this antipsorics are called for because*, when syphilis has advanced so far, psora has usually got mixed with it (Kent). If either psora or sycosis is active when syphilis is taken the syphilis usually suppresses the other miasm, and when after a period of antisyphilitic remedies the disease becomes latent the symptoms of the sycosis or psora begin and must be treated by their corresponding remedies until they in turn become latent. The syphilis may again become active, and this alternation of the different miasms may go on for a time before the patient is thoroughly cured.

This alternation of the miasms is very important, because antipsoric remedies, such as *Sulph.*, *Calc.* and *Graph*, are more likely to do harm than good if given while the syphilis is active. (Kent).

When syphilis has progressed till gummatous formation have been produced round the anus, in periosteum and in the brain, *Sulph.*, if given, will suppurate these and thus make the patient worse. I have seen it suppurate the soft palate away when I did not know he had syphilis. You may have to give at once *Merc. or Merc-c.* To stop action of the *Sulph.* (Kent)

SYCOSIS

There are two forms of gonorrhea, the acute and the chronic. There is also a psoric catarrhal form or urethritis. The acute is much the most common form and its suppression does not lead to constitutional symptoms. [Kent. *Journal of Homeopathics*, April 1899.]

The chronic form begins in exactly the same way as the acute and to all outward appearance the discharge is the same [Kent]. As long as this chronic form permitted to discharge freely no constitutional symptoms appear, thus markedly differing from syphilis. [Kent, *Med. Adv.*, Nov. 1888]

The second manifestation of sycosis is the figwart which is usually soft, sensitive, easily bleeding, red, with an offensive, sweet smell. Sometimes the warts are smooth, red, shining. As long as these warts are allowed to remain undisturbed no constitutional symptoms appear. It is to be remembered that both the discharge and warts may be suppressed by the continual use of inappropriate homeopathic remedies.

The first constitutional symptom of sycosis is the rheumatism, which may not appear for some months after the disappearance of the primary manifestation. This rheumatism is very similar to that caused by *Rhus-t.* but that remedy only palliates as it is not an anti-sycotic.

The order in which the other manifestation appear in not well known, but amongst the chief are orchitis, red phthisis and many affections of the female genitals. It also causes asthma, which is apt. to be aggravated in warm moist weather or in the spring.

According to Kent spasmodic asthma is almost invariably sycotic, especially if hereditary, and remedies like *Spong, Ip., Carb- v., Bry.* and *Ars.* only palliate. One of its latest and most marked manifestations is a peculiar anemia characterized by a waxy, shining, greenish-grey appearance of the face, with hollow cheeks and voice.

Sycosis, like syphilis, can, as a rule only be taken once, according to Kent, and in these cases of repeated gonorrhea only one was real or sycotic. In exception to this, a man in the last stage of the constitutional state, can take gonorrhea in the first stage and go through the whole course, and woman who has the anemic state would, if exposed, get the discharge (Kent)

Sycosis, like syphilis, is always taken at the stage it has arrived at in the person from whom it is taken and consequently many women only have it at the anemic stage.

When we pave to treat a case of constitutional sycosis we must choose our remedy in accordance with the symptoms that are present, and as a rule, this will be found to be one of the anti-sycotics. At times, however, we may have to go outside the list of known anti-sycotics, for at present it is far from complete. In these cases of constitutional sycosis, when the suitable remedy removes one group, the next will appear, probably calling for another remedy, and this process will have to be continued from stage to stage until we have taken the patient through all he has formerly experienced, but the stages will appear in the opposite order to that in which they first came. In advanced cases it may take two or three years before we can bring back the primary manifestations whether that was a gonorrhea, a rheumatism, or a catarrh. If, when we restore the original gonorrhea, it fails to remain for a length of time. It shows a want of reaction on the part of the patient and the cure will be doubtful.

Mercury and *Sulphur* seldom do anything but harm in advanced sycosis, though often indicated in the stage of discharge. It is rarely possible to cure old sycotic strictures by medicines, and it can only be done when the remedy sets up an acute urethritis with the return of the original gonorrhea.

If the convalescence from acute disease is delayed we must not invariably regard the cause to be psora, but find out what miasm is present and give the corresponding antipsoric, antisyphilitic or anti-sycotic (Kent).

A marked similarity between the symptoms of sycosis and those produced by vaccination led Boenninghausen and others to regard them as indentical but Kent does not believe this to be correct.

Ordinary *gleet* lingering for months is *not* always indicative of sycosis, but often of psora and analogous to catarrh from any other mucous membrane. (Kent)

It is worthy of notice that many remedies have a decided curative action upon the gonorrheal discharge; but are not known to have cured warty cases or to have developed a suppressed discharge. It may be they are only gonorrhea remedies and may cure the discharge and not sycosis. Any condition driven from the urethra my produce inflammation of the testicle, not necessarily sycotic. Remedies for the suppression of the discharge are, therefore, not necessarily anti-sycotic. (Kent)

INDEX